I0429619

TABLE OF CONTENTS

Milk & Milk Products

Type	Quantity	Calories
Full-fat milk	1 cup	150
Low fat milk (1%)	1 cup	102
Cow's milk	1 cup	157
Goat milk	1 cup	264
Sweetened Condensed Milk "cans"	28 g	123
Full cream milk powder	Half a cup	635
Skim milk powder	Half a cup	435
Full-fat chocolate milk	1 cup	208
Strawberry Milk	1 cup	244
Cheddar cheese slices	Slice, 28 gm	114
Feta cheese	28 g	75
Finuta cheese	25 g	110
Gouda cheese	28 g	101
Mozzarella cheese	28 g	80
Kraft Cheese "cups"	28 g	80
Edam cheese	28 g	98
Blue cheese	28 g	104
Harafati cheese	28 g	116
Mascarpone cheese	28 g	128
Ricotta cheese "whole milk"	Half a cup	216
Ricotta cheese, partly skim milk	Half a cup	171

Parmesan cheese	28 g	130
Camembert cheese	28 g	86
Cottage cheese	100 g	99
Akkawi cheese	100 g	289
Kashkaval cheese	100 g	404
Halloumi cheese	100 g	363
Cream focused	1 spoon	52
Cream Medium	1 spoon	37
Rob "yogurt" full-fat	1 spoon	141
Rob "yogurt" skim	1 spoon	114
Brick	155 g	105
Clabber	1 cup	99
Vanilla ice cream 10% fat	Half a cup	135

Ice Cream

Vanilla	1 ball	240
Cocoa	1 ball	280
Strawberries	1 ball	220

Drinks & Juices

Type	Quantity	Calories
Apple juice	Half a cup	60
Apricot juice, canned	Half a cup	72
Grape juice, canned	Half a cup	78
Lemon juice canned	Spoon to eat	3
Fresh orange juice	Half a cup	59
Canned orange juice	Half a cup	52
Grapefruit juice, canned local	Half a cup	58
Grapefruit juice, unsweetened	Half a cup	47
Canned peach juice	Half a cup	67
Canned pear juice	Half a cup	75
Canned pineapple juice	Half a cup	70
Canned tomato juice	Half a cup	21
Canned juice Islands	Half a cup	49
Guava juice	One cup	175
Mango juice	One cup	110
Vimto juice	One cup	165

Hot Drinks

Nescafe coffee without sugar	Teaspoon	5
Instant coffee without caffeine	Teaspoon	5
Tea without sugar	One cup	1
American coffee	One cup	5

Soft Drinks

Pepsi-Cola	240 ml cup	100
Diet Pepsi-Cola	240 ml cup	0.00
Seven Up	240 ml cup	90
Sprite	240 ml cup	96
Fanta	240 ml cup	119
Coca-Cola	240 ml cup	97
Diet Coca-Cola	240 ml cup	1.00
Cream soda	240 ml cup	126
Drink grape gas	240 ml cup	107

Luncheon and Sausage Meat

Type	Quantity	Calories
Beef	Approx. 42 g	142
Pastrami - turkey	28 g	40
Pepperoni beef	28 g	141
Salami - turkey	28 g	56
Salami - beef	28 g	72
Mortadella - beef	28 g	47
Bologna sausage		
Turkey	28 g	57
Beef	28 g	88
Frankfurter		
Turkey	42 g	102
Chicken meat	42 g	116

Eggs

Type	Quantity	Calories
Egg whites, (fresh or iced)	One, big	17
Fresh egg yolk	One, big	59
Full cook boiled eggs	One, big	79
Fried eggs	One, big	91
Omelet	One, big	92
Omelet with cheese and vegetables	113 g	252
Duck eggs	One, big	130
Goose eggs	One, big	267
Turkey eggs	One, big	135
Quail eggs	One, big	14

Nuts & Legumes

Type	Quantity	Calories
Nuts	Half a cup, 60 g	380
Almonds, dry	Quarter a cup	209
Cashew, roasted, dry	28 g	160
Cashew, roasted, oily	28 g	165
Nuts, roasted, dry	28 g	170
Hazelnut, roasted, oily	28 g	176
Lentils, whole, green	Half a cup	215
Lentils, cooked	One cup	210

Oils & Fats

Type	Quantity	Calories
Margarine	1 Tablespoon	105
Olive oil	1 Tablespoon	120
Sunflower oil	1 Tablespoon	120
Sheep fat	1 Tablespoon	114
Vegetable oil	1 Tablespoon	126
Beef fat	1 Tablespoon	125
Butter	1 Tablespoon	36
Corn oil	1 Tablespoon	120

Fresh Fruits

Type	Quantity	Calories
Apples	Medium, 140 g	81
Apricot	Medium, 30 g	17
Banana	Medium, 100 g	105
Fig	One, 40 g	37
Grapefruit	Half	38
Cherries	10 beads	49
Avocado	Half	162
Grapes	Half a cup	53
Guava	One, 85 g	45
Kiwi	One, 76 g	46
Mango	Half, 85 g	68
Orange	One, 110 g	62
Papaya	Medium	117
Peach	One, 85 g	37
Pear	Medium, 170 g	98
Pineapple	Slice, 82 g	42
Plum	One, 60 g	36
Pomegranate	Medium, 150 g	110
Nectarine	Medium, 142 g	67
Watermelon	Piece, 100 g	26
Melon	Piece, 100 g	33

Strawberries	Half a cup	23
Tangerine	One, 85 g	37
Blueberry	One cup	122
Rutab/ripe dates	10 beads	150
Loquat	100 g	49
Plum	100 g	52
Lemon	One, 60 g	17
Sweet Lemon	Fruit size	53
Black berry	One cup	117
Nabq (rhamnus)	30 beads	9
Quince	Medium	60
Tamarind	Half a cup	82

Canned Fruits

Type	Quantity	Calories
Canned apricots (with sugar syrup)	Half a cup	111
Fruit salad (with sugar syrup)	Half a cup	94
Canned cherry (with thick sugar syrup)	Half a cup	107
Canned peaches (with sugar syrup)	Half a cup	95
Canned pear with (with sugar syrup)	Half a cup	94
Canned pineapple (with sugar syrup)	Half a cup	100

Dried Fruits

Type	Quantity	Calories
Dried dates	One	26
Dried figs	100 g	288
Raisins	Half a cup	109
Dried plum	Half a cup	113
Dried Apricots	Half a cup	169

Spices

Type	Quantity	Calories
Cardamom	1 teaspoon	7
Dried hot red pepper	3 teaspoons	13
Cinnamon	1 teaspoon	7
Cloves	1 teaspoon	6
Latency	1 teaspoon	6
Ginger "powder"	1 teaspoon	1
Ginger root	One, medium	20
Nutmeg "powder"	1 teaspoon	9
Black pepper	1 teaspoon	8

Red Meat

Type	Quantity	Calories
Lamb shoulder, cooked with fat	63 g	220
Lamb shoulder, cooked without fat	48 g	135
Lamb thigh, roasted with fat	85 g	205
Lamb thigh, roasted without fat	73 g	140
Lamb rib, grilled without fat	85 g	200
Lamb rib, grilled with fat	85 g	307
Beef, chest, cooked	85 g	189
Beef shoulder, without fat	85 g	183
Beef, minced and cooked	85 g	245
Shawarma, only meat	85 g	317
Beef steak without fat	85 g	174
Tekkah	85 g	133
Kebab	85 g	226
Kubba, stuffed	85 g	281
Slices without fat	85 g	182
Cow heart, cooked	85 g	148
Cow kidney, cooked	85 g	122
Cow tongue, cooked	85 g	241

Vegetables

Type	Quantity	Calories
Carrot	Medium, 60 g	31
Carrot, cooked	Half a cup	35
Cauliflower, cooked	Half a cup	15
Cauliflower, uncooked	Half a cup	12
Cucumbers, chopped	Half a cup	7
Fried eggplant	Half a cup	100
Eggplant, cooked	Half a cup	13
Green beans, cooked	Half a cup	20
Green beans, canned	Half a cup	25
Cabbage, cooked	Half a cup	16
Cabbage, uncooked	Half a cup	8
Celery	Half a cup	10
Corn	One, medium	77
Mushrooms, fresh	Half a cup	9
Mushroom, canned	Half a cup	19
Lettuce	Half a cup	4
Mixed vegetables (a variety of vegetables cooked together)	Half a cup	54
Okra, cooked and chopped	Half a cup	25
Fresh onions, chopped	Half a cup	27
Green onions, chopped	Half a cup	16
Green peas, cooked	Half a cup	67

Peppers, chopped	Half a cup	12
Hot pepper	One, 30 g	18
Baked potato, with the peel	195 g	220
Baked potato, without the peel	195 g	162
Fried potato	10 pieces, 42 g	158
Shalgam kale, boiled	Half a cup	14
Watercress	Half a cup	2
Squash	Half a cup	41
Red rweid radish	10 grains, 40 g	7
Red rweid radish, leaves	10 leaves, medium	9
Chopped spinach	Half a cup	6
Zucchini, chopped and cooked	Half a cup	18
Sweet potatoes, mashed	Half a cup	111
Red tomatoes	One, medium	26
Green beans	One cup	73
Beet	One cup	46
Cabbage	One cup	73
Leek	1 Spoon, minced	1
Coriander	1 package	97
Fenugreek, leaves	1 package	25
Garlic	5 pieces of garlic peeled	7
Grape leaves	1 cup	146

Mint	Package, medium	84
Black olives	10 grains, medium	95
Green olives	10 grains, medium	66
Parsley	1 cup, minced	34
Parsley	Package, medium	25
White rweid radishes	Package, medium	58
Spinach	1 Cup, chopped	14
Zucchini	1 cup, chopped	31
Zucchini	One, medium	40
Basil	100 g	50
Boil	100 g	32
Legume	100 g	32
Sugar-cane	100 g	82

Grains

Type	Quantity	Calories
Bread, cereals	100 g	17
Lebanese bread	Quarter of a loaf	70
Oven bread, Iranian	Quarter of a loaf	79
Whole wheat bread	One, 50 g	130
Manaqich (bread with thyme)	One, 75 g	208
Sammon	One, 75 g	209
Rusk (cake)	50 g	150
Pasta with sauce	Small, 130 g	190
Corn flakes	Cup, 25 g	95
French bread	Quarter of a loaf, 115 g	333
Plain biscuits	4 pieces, 55 g	178
White rice, cooked (long grain)	Half a cup	131
Brown toast	A slice	61
Plain white toast	A slice	64
Spaghetti, cooked or pasta	Half a cup	99
Spaghetti, cooked with minced meat and tomato	Half a cup	110
Lasagna with meat sauce	Half a cup	154
	One cup	672

Barley		
Pasta	One cup	344
Cornstarch	One cup	471
Rice, uncooked	One cup	675
Rice powder	One cup	354
Vermicelli (balaleet)	One cup	99
Bulgur (groats, crushed)	One cup	613
Wheat	One cup	485
Jabati (Indian bread)	One, medium	225

Meat & Chicken

Type	Quantity	Calories
Chicken leg (hip), without skin, grilled	85 g	167
Chicken leg (hip), with skin, grilled	85 g	223
Chicken breast, without skin, grilled	Half a breast	142
Chicken breast, with skin, grilled	Half a breast	193
Chicken breast, without skin, fried	Half a breast	161
Chicken wings, with skin, grilled	1 wing "35.5 g"	99
Chicken pieces, vacuum, fried	6 pieces "104 g"	290
Chicken gizzards, fried	85 g	238
Chicken livers, cooked	85 g	135
Duck meat, without skin, roasted	85 g	173
Kinds of Turkey Meat		
Red dark meat, without skin	85 g	161
Red dark meat, with skin	85 g	190
Red light meat, meat without skin	85 g	135
Red light meat, meat with skin	85 g	169

Fish and Shellfish

Type	Quantity	Calories
Sardines, canned in oil	28 g	58
Anchovies, canned in oil	21 g	42
Tuna, canned in water	85 g	104
Tuna, canned in oil	85 g	169
Smoked salmon	85 g	99
Grilled Fish	85 g	136
Fish fried with rusk	3 pieces, 85 g	228
Shrimp fried with rusk	85 g	206
Crab, canned	85 g	84
Shrimp, cooked	85 g	83
Oyster, uncooked	28 g	23
Oysters, fried	28 g	46
Oysters, fried with rusk	85 g	84
Caviar, black or red	1 tablespoon	40

Legumes

Type	Quantity	Calories
Beans, boiled	One cup	187
Dry beans	One cup	349
Beans	Half a cup	37
Chickpeas, boiled	Half a cup	269
Flour	One cup	339
Lentil	Half a cup	192
Nuts mixed with roasted and dry peanuts	28 g	170
Mixed nuts roasted in oil	28 g	175
Sunflower seeds, roasted and dry	28 g	170
Sunflower seed, roasted in oil	28 g	175
Pistachios, dry and roasted	Half a cup	357
Peanuts, dry and roasted	28 g	165
Peanuts, roasted in oil	28 g	170
Peanut butter	Spoon 16 g	95
Roasted chestnut	28 g	44
Coconut	28 g	100
Grated coconut	28 g	59
Roasted pumpkin seeds	28 g	127
Dried watermelon seeds	28 g	158
Circuit pills	28 g	102.2
Sesame	28 g	174.16
Pine	28 g	172.7

NOTES

NOTES

NOTES

NOTES

NOTES

www.ingramcontent.com/pod-product-compliance
Lightning Source LLC
Chambersburg PA
CBHW072014280526
45788CB00005B/2036